Her Health on a Plate: A Woman Centric Cookbook

Nourishing Every Woman:
Empowering Lives Through
Wholesome Culinary Choices

Daniel C. Wright

Table of Contents

Introduction

Her Health on a Plate: A Woman Centric Cookbook" invites you on a culinary journey tailored to celebrate and nourish women's well-being. In a world where nutrition is pivotal, this cookbook goes beyond mere recipes, intertwining the art of cooking with a deep understanding of women's unique health needs. With women at the heart of its culinary canvas, this cookbook is a testament to the power of mindful eating.This exceptional collection of recipes is meticulously crafted to address the nutritional requirements specific to women at various life stages. From adolescence to adulthood, pregnancy to menopause, each section offers delicious and balanced meals that cater to the distinct needs of a woman's body. The cookbook delves into the symbiotic relationship between food and women's health, emphasizing ingredients rich in essential nutrients like iron, calcium, and omega-3 fatty acids.Beyond nourishment, "Her Health on a Plate" embraces the idea that food is a source of joy and empowerment. The recipes are not only designed for optimal health but also to delight the palate, ensuring that women relish every bite. The cookbook's approach goes beyond the conventional, introducing innovative and culturally diverse recipes that cater to various tastes and preferences.In addition to the delectable recipes, the cookbook incorporates valuable insights from nutritionists, health experts, and chefs who specialize in women's health. This holistic approach provides readers with a comprehensive understanding of the nutritional science behind each dish, empowering them to make informed choices for their well-being."Her Health on a Plate" is more than a cookbook; it's a companion on the journey to vibrant health for women. With its thoughtful curation of recipes, nutritional expertise, and celebration of the joy of cooking, this cookbook is a testament to the philosophy that good health begins on one's plate. Embrace the fusion of flavor and well-being as you embark on a culinary adventure tailored for women, ensuring that every meal is a step towards a healthier, happier you.

Chapter One
Nourishing the Body:
Understanding Women's
Unique Nutritional Needs

Nourishing the Body - Understanding Women's Unique Nutritional NeedsIn the intricate tapestry of women's health, the first chapter delves into the crucial aspect of nourishing the body. Recognizing and addressing the unique nutritional needs of women is pivotal for promoting overall well-being and preventing a myriad of health issues.The chapter commences with an exploration of the physiological disparities between men and women, shedding light on how these differences influence nutritional requirements. From hormonal fluctuations to reproductive health, understanding these nuances is essential in tailoring dietary recommendations to women's distinct needs.An emphasis is placed on the role of key nutrients such as iron, calcium, and folate, which play vital roles in women's health.

Iron, for instance, is crucial for combating the risk of anemia, a prevalent concern among women. Calcium, essential for bone health, becomes even more significant during various life stages, such as pregnancy and menopause. Folate, a B-vitamin, assumes a pivotal role in preventing neural tube defects during pregnancy.The chapter also navigates through the labyrinth of women's dietary preferences and challenges, acknowledging the socio-cultural factors that can impact nutritional choices. From addressing the prevalence of dieting trends to promoting body positivity, the narrative aims to foster a holistic understanding of women's relationships with food.Furthermore, the chapter highlights the significance of lifestyle factors, including physical activity and stress management, in conjunction with nutrition. These elements are intertwined in the intricate dance of promoting women's health and must be considered in tandem for comprehensive well-being.By the conclusion of Chapter One, readers gain a foundational understanding of the intricate interplay between women's unique physiological aspects and their nutritional requirements. Armed with this knowledge, individuals are better equipped to make informed choices, fostering a path towards optimal health and vitality for women at every stage of life

Chapter Two
Empowering Choices: The Role of Diet in Women's Health

Empowering Choices: The Role of Diet in Women's HealthIn the intricate tapestry of women's health, Chapter Two delves into the profound impact of dietary choices. Acknowledging that what we consume plays a pivotal role in overall well-being, this chapter is a beacon of empowerment, guiding women towards informed decisions that nurture their bodies.The chapter begins by unraveling the intricate relationship between nutrition and women's health. It illuminates the physiological nuances unique to women, emphasizing how dietary habits can influence hormonal balance, reproductive health, and overall vitality. Readers are encouraged to view their dietary choices not merely as a routine but as a conscious act that shapes their journey towards optimal health.A cornerstone of this chapter is the exploration of nutrient-rich foods that are particularly beneficial for women. From essential vitamins to minerals crucial for bone health, the narrative unfolds the nutritional elements necessary to fortify the female body. Practical tips and accessible meal plans are woven into the fabric of the chapter, ensuring that readers can seamlessly incorporate these empowering choices into their daily lives.Furthermore, the chapter demystifies prevalent myths surrounding diet and women's health. By debunking misconceptions and fostering a science-backed understanding of nutrition, it equips women to make informed decisions tailored to their unique needs. The narrative also addresses the societal pressures and unrealistic standards often associated with women's diets, promoting a holistic approach that values health over unrealistic ideals.As the chapter progresses, it explores the intersectionality of diet, mental health, and emotional well-being. Highlighting the intricate connection between what we eat and how we feel, it advocates for a balanced approach that nurtures both the body and mind. By fostering mindfulness around food choices, women are empowered to cultivate a harmonious relationship with their bodies.In conclusion, Chapter Two serves as a roadmap for women to navigate the complex terrain of dietary choices. It empowers them to make informed decisions that resonate with their unique physiology, fostering a holistic approach to health and well-being. Through knowledge, practical insights, and a celebration of individuality, this chapter guides women towards a path of empowerment and vitality.

Chapter Three
Breakfasts for Balance:
Energize Your Day

Breakfasts for Balance: Energize Your DayIn the pursuit of a healthy and balanced lifestyle, the significance of breakfast cannot be overstated. Chapter Three delves into the realm of morning nourishment, offering insights and practical tips to energize your day right from the start. Aptly titled "Breakfasts for Balance," this chapter serves as a nutritional compass, guiding readers towards choices that fuel both body and mind.The chapter opens with a compelling exploration of the physiological benefits of a well-rounded breakfast. From kickstarting metabolism to enhancing cognitive function, the research-backed evidence underscores the pivotal role breakfast plays in setting a positive tone for the day. As readers delve into the content, they will discover a myriad of breakfast options tailored to meet diverse tastes and dietary preferences.A highlight of this chapter is the emphasis on balance – a key principle that resonates throughout the entire book. Whether you're a fan of savory or sweet, a dedicated carnivore or a plant-based enthusiast, there's a breakfast recommendation designed to harmonize with your individual needs. From nutrient-dense smoothie bowls bursting with antioxidants to protein-packed egg variations, the chapter's recipes are not only delicious but also meticulously crafted to provide a symphony of essential nutrients.Practicality is a cornerstone of the breakfast recommendations outlined in Chapter Three. Recognizing the time constraints of modern life, the chapter introduces time-efficient options that do not compromise on nutritional value. Quick and easy recipes, make-ahead options, and on-the-go breakfast ideas ensure that the commitment to a balanced morning meal seamlessly integrates into daily routines.As readers navigate through the chapter, they will find not just a collection of recipes but a comprehensive guide to crafting breakfasts that transcend mere sustenance. Breakfasts for Balance is an empowering resource that fosters a deeper understanding of the symbiotic relationship between food and well-being, paving the way for a revitalized and energized start to each day.

Chapter Four
Lunches with Love: Fueling Your Afternoon

Lunches with Love: Fueling Your AfternoonIn the bustling rhythm of our daily lives, the importance of a well-balanced lunch often gets overshadowed by hectic schedules and looming deadlines. "Lunches with Love: Fueling Your Afternoon," the pivotal Chapter Four of our guide, seeks to shift this narrative. Acknowledging lunch not merely as a necessity but as a source of nourishment and vitality, this chapter delves into the art of crafting lunches that transcend the mundane and truly fuel your afternoons with love.The chapter opens with a reflection on the impact of a thoughtful lunch on overall well-being. By exploring the intersection of nutrition, mood, and productivity, readers gain insights into the profound effects a wholesome midday meal can have on their physical and mental states. It serves as a reminder that nourishing the body isn't just about meeting caloric needs but fostering a harmonious connection between mind and body.With an emphasis on variety and balance, the chapter unfolds a plethora of lunch ideas catering to different dietary preferences and constraints. From vibrant salads bursting with nutrients to hearty protein-packed bowls, the recipes provided are not only delicious but also designed to sustain energy levels throughout the afternoon. This section acts as a practical guide for readers seeking to break free from monotonous lunch routines and explore the rich tapestry of flavors available to them.Beyond the culinary aspect, "Lunches with Love" encourages readers to embrace mindful eating practices. By savoring each bite and taking moments of respite during the lunch break, individuals can cultivate a deeper connection with their food, fostering a sense of gratitude and joy.Incorporating expert insights on nutrition, the chapter also addresses common misconceptions about what constitutes a healthy lunch. It dispels myths, offering evidence-based information that empowers readers to make informed choices aligned with their health goals.In essence, Chapter Four serves as a compass for transforming lunchtime into a ritual of self-care. By infusing love into our midday meals, we not only nourish our bodies but also cultivate a positive relationship with food, paving the way for heightened well-being and sustained productivity throughout the day.

Chapter Five: Dinners for Wellness: Delicious and Nutrient-Packed

Chapter Six
Snacks for Sustained Energy: Smart Bites for Every Craving

Snacks for Sustained Energy: Smart Bites for Every CravingIn the quest for sustained energy throughout the day, Chapter Six of our comprehensive guide delves into the art of snacking wisely. Titled "Snacks for Sustained Energy: Smart Bites for Every Craving," this chapter is a treasure trove of insights and practical tips to keep you fueled and focused.The chapter begins by emphasizing the importance of strategic snacking in maintaining optimal energy levels. Whether you're battling the mid-morning slump or the afternoon lull, the right snacks can make a significant difference. Readers are introduced to a variety of smart bites designed to cater to every craving, ensuring a delightful and nutritious snacking experience.From protein-packed options to wholesome carbs and nutrient-dense treats, the chapter explores a diverse range of snacks tailored to different dietary preferences and needs. Whether you're a fitness enthusiast seeking a post-workout boost or someone looking for brain-boosting snacks to enhance productivity, you'll find a plethora of options to suit your taste and lifestyle.Readers will discover easy-to-follow recipes and snack ideas that can be effortlessly incorporated into their daily routines. The emphasis is not just on energy but on sustained energy, promoting snacks that provide a gradual release of nutrients to keep you going throughout the day.To further enhance the reader's understanding, the chapter includes expert insights on the science behind sustained energy snacks. Understanding how certain nutrients contribute to prolonged vitality empowers individuals to make informed choices that align with their specific health and wellness goals.In conclusion, Chapter Six serves as a comprehensive guide to navigating the world of snacks for sustained energy. Whether you're a seasoned health enthusiast or just beginning your journey towards mindful eating, this chapter equips you with the knowledge and inspiration needed to make smart snack choices that support your overall well-being.

Chapter Seven
Sweet Treats, Smart Sweets: Indulging Healthily

Sweet Treats, Smart Sweets: Indulging HealthilyIn the pursuit of a balanced and wholesome lifestyle, Chapter Seven of our wellness journey delves into the delightful realm of "Sweet Treats, Smart Sweets." This chapter is a compass guiding us towards the realm of guilt-free indulgence, where the joy of savoring delectable treats meets the wisdom of mindful consumption.Gone are the days when the word "sweet" was synonymous with an avalanche of sugar and regret. Our exploration begins with the understanding that indulging in treats doesn't have to be a compromise on health. Enter the era of smart sweets – a thoughtful selection of delicious confections that cater to both the palate and well-being.This chapter is a revelation of innovative recipes and smart choices that redefine our relationship with sweets. Learn the art of crafting desserts with alternative sweeteners, harnessing the natural sweetness of fruits, and incorporating nutrient-dense ingredients. Discover the alchemy of transforming traditional favorites into health-conscious delights without sacrificing taste.We navigate through the maze of sugar substitutes, shedding light on options that don't just sweeten but contribute to better health. Dive into the world of stevia, monk fruit, and other plant-based alternatives that make your treats not only sweeter but smarter.Moreover, the chapter doesn't just stop at recipes. It provides insights into the psychology of cravings and how to maintain a balanced approach to satisfy the sweet tooth. Explore portion control, mindful eating practices, and strategies to overcome the allure of sugary temptations.By the end of this chapter, you'll not only have a repertoire of mouthwatering recipes but also a newfound appreciation for the art of crafting smart sweets. Indulging healthily becomes a joyous celebration, where each bite is a harmonious blend of flavor and well-being. So, let's embark on this flavorful journey, savoring the sweetness of life without compromising our commitment to health and vitality.

Chapter Eight: Culinary Medicine: Foods for Hormonal Harmony

Culinary Medicine: Foods for Hormonal HarmonyIn the intricate symphony of the human body, hormones play a pivotal role in orchestrating various physiological processes. Chapter Eight delves into the realm of Culinary Medicine, shedding light on the profound impact that specific foods can have on hormonal balance. The chapter explores the intersection of nutrition and hormonal harmony, offering a holistic approach to well-being.At the core of this culinary exploration are foods that exert a direct influence on hormonal regulation. From enhancing insulin sensitivity to supporting thyroid function, the chapter meticulously unravels the connections between dietary choices and hormonal health. It emphasizes the importance of a well-balanced diet rich in nutrients that are essential for the production and regulation of hormones.Readers are guided through a gastronomic journey, discovering the power of certain foods in promoting hormonal equilibrium. Whether it's incorporating omega-3 fatty acids for brain health or embracing phytoestrogen-rich options for reproductive well-being, the chapter provides practical insights into crafting a hormone-friendly menu.Furthermore, the chapter elucidates the impact of lifestyle factors on hormonal health, underscoring the significance of mindful eating and stress management. It explores how culinary choices can act as potent tools in mitigating the effects of chronic stress on hormonal balance, fostering resilience in the face of modern-day challenges.Through evidence-backed research and culinary wisdom, the chapter offers a roadmap for individuals seeking to optimize their hormonal health through dietary interventions. It advocates for a personalized approach, recognizing the uniqueness of each individual's hormonal profile and tailoring nutritional strategies accordingly.In summary, Chapter Eight serves as a beacon for those navigating the intricate landscape of hormonal harmony. By weaving together the science of nutrition and the art of cooking, it empowers readers to embrace a culinary medicine approach that not only delights the taste buds but also nurtures the delicate dance of hormones within the body.

Chapter Nine
A Culinary Journey through Women's Wellness: Recipes from Around the World

A Culinary Journey through Women's Wellness: Recipes from Around the World" is a flavorful exploration of global cuisines that prioritize women's health. This chapter transcends borders, bringing together a diverse array of recipes that celebrate the intersection of culture and well-being.The culinary journey starts with a section dedicated to Mediterranean delights, renowned for their heart-healthy ingredients. From Greek salads bursting with vibrant vegetables to Spanish paella rich in antioxidants, these recipes embody the essence of the Mediterranean lifestyle, promoting longevity and vitality.Continuing eastward, the chapter delves into the nourishing traditions of Asian cuisine. Japanese miso soup, Chinese herbal teas, and Indian turmeric-infused dishes showcase the medicinal properties of spices and herbs, offering a holistic approach to women's wellness rooted in centuries-old practices.The flavors of Africa take center stage in the next section, highlighting nutrient-dense ingredients that contribute to overall health. From Moroccan chickpea stew to South African rooibos-infused desserts, the recipes draw inspiration from the continent's diverse culinary heritage, emphasizing the importance of balance and variety in one's diet.The Latin American portion of the chapter is a vibrant tapestry of colors and flavors, featuring dishes that combine indigenous ingredients with modern nutritional knowledge. Quinoa salads, Brazilian acai bowls, and Mexican avocado-based recipes showcase the richness of the region's culinary landscape, reflecting a commitment to both taste and well-being.Closing the culinary journey, the chapter concludes with a fusion of global influences, illustrating how different cuisines can harmoniously contribute to women's wellness. The recipes are not only delicious but also designed to support physical health and mental well-being.In essence, Chapter Nine is a testament to the idea that a well-rounded and culturally diverse diet is integral to women's overall wellness. Through these recipes, readers are invited to savor the world's culinary treasures while nurturing their health and embracing the wisdom passed down through generations.

Chapter Ten
Mindful Eating: Enhancing the Connection between Food and Well-being

Chapter Ten of the book explores the concept of mindful eating and its profound impact on the connection between food and overall well-being. Mindful eating is a practice rooted in mindfulness, encouraging individuals to pay full attention to the sensory experiences associated with eating. This chapter delves into the transformative effects of adopting a mindful approach to consuming food.The author begins by emphasizing the importance of being present during meals, highlighting how the act of eating can be elevated from a mere routine to a mindful experience. Through various anecdotes and research findings, the chapter elucidates the link between conscious eating and improved mental and physical health.Mindful eating involves cultivating awareness of hunger and satiety cues, savoring the flavors and textures of food, and recognizing the impact of emotions on eating habits. The chapter delves into practical techniques, such as mindful breathing and slowing down the pace of eating, to facilitate a deeper connection with the act of nourishing the body.Furthermore, the author explores the psychological aspects of mindful eating, discussing how it can contribute to a healthier relationship with food. By being attuned to the body's signals and breaking free from automatic eating patterns, individuals can make more informed choices that align with their nutritional needs.The chapter also addresses the potential benefits of mindful eating in addressing issues like overeating, emotional eating, and unhealthy dietary habits. It provides readers with a roadmap to cultivate mindfulness in their eating practices, offering practical tips and exercises to integrate this approach into their daily lives.In conclusion, Chapter Ten underscores the significance of mindful eating as a powerful tool for enhancing the connection between food and well-being. By embracing a more intentional and conscious approach to eating, individuals can foster a harmonious relationship with food that contributes to their overall health and happiness.

Chapter Eleven
Fitness Fuel: Recipes to Support an Active Lifestyle

Fitness Fuel: Recipes to Support an Active LifestyleIn the journey towards a healthier and more active lifestyle, the importance of nutrition cannot be overstated. Chapter Eleven of our comprehensive guide focuses on "Fitness Fuel," providing a collection of recipes meticulously crafted to support and enhance your physical endeavors.The chapter kicks off with a fundamental understanding of the relationship between nutrition and an active lifestyle. It delves into the specific dietary needs of individuals engaged in various levels of physical activity, from casual exercisers to dedicated athletes. Readers gain insights into the essential nutrients that fuel energy, aid recovery, and promote overall well-being.The recipes featured in this chapter are designed with a dual purpose – to be delicious and to provide the necessary sustenance for optimum performance. From pre-workout snacks to post-exercise meals, each recipe is a fusion of taste and nutritional value. Whether you're preparing for a high-intensity training session or looking to replenish your energy stores after a workout, the chapter offers a diverse range of options to suit every palate.Highlights include nutrient-packed smoothie bowls bursting with antioxidants, protein-rich power bars for on-the-go energy, and savory post-workout meals that strike the perfect balance between carbs, proteins, and healthy fats. Each recipe comes with a breakdown of its nutritional content, empowering readers to make informed choices tailored to their fitness goals.Beyond the kitchen, Chapter Eleven extends its guidance to hydration strategies, emphasizing the crucial role of water in sustaining peak performance. Practical tips on timing meals, portion control, and adapting recipes to individual dietary preferences ensure that readers can seamlessly incorporate these fitness-fueling recipes into their daily lives.By the end of this chapter, readers will not only have a repertoire of delicious and nutritious recipes but also a comprehensive understanding of how to optimize their diet to support an active lifestyle. "Fitness Fuel" is not just a culinary journey; it's a roadmap to harnessing the power of food to elevate your fitness journey to new heights.

Chapter Twelve
Herbs and Spices for Women's Health: Beyond Flavor

Herbs and Spices for Women's Health: Beyond Flavor" delves into the transformative power of herbs and spices in promoting women's well-being beyond mere culinary delights. In this insightful exploration, the author unravels the age-old secrets of nature's pharmacy, revealing how herbs and spices can contribute to women's health in multifaceted ways.The chapter opens with a historical perspective, tracing the traditional uses of herbs and spices in various cultures to address women's specific health concerns. From menstrual discomfort to hormonal balance, the author draws on the wisdom of ancient herbal remedies, providing a rich tapestry of knowledge that transcends time.The narrative then seamlessly transitions to a modern understanding of the science behind these botanical wonders. Scientific studies and research findings are presented to substantiate the efficacy of herbs and spices in addressing contemporary women's health issues. Readers are guided through the biochemical intricacies that make herbs and spices potent allies in supporting reproductive health, managing stress, and mitigating common ailments.A significant portion of the chapter is dedicated to practical applications, offering readers a comprehensive guide on incorporating herbs and spices into their daily lives. From teas and tinctures to culinary masterpieces, the author provides recipes and suggestions that empower women to harness the therapeutic potential of these natural wonders.The holistic approach of the chapter extends beyond the physical aspects of health, delving into the emotional and mental well-being of women. The author explores how certain herbs and spices can positively impact mood, stress levels, and overall mental resilience.In conclusion, Chapter Twelve serves as a beacon of knowledge, illuminating the transformative role of herbs and spices in promoting women's health beyond flavor. With a harmonious blend of ancient wisdom and modern science, readers are empowered to embrace these botanical allies on their journey to holistic well-being.

Chapter Thirteen: Celebrating Womanhood: Special Occasion Recipes

Celebrating Womanhood: Special Occasion RecipesIn this enchanting chapter, we delve into the art of celebrating womanhood through a curated collection of special occasion recipes. Each dish is a testament to the strength, grace, and resilience inherent in every woman, making it a fitting tribute to the essence of femininity.The chapter opens with a celebration of milestones, offering recipes tailored for events that mark significant moments in a woman's life. From birthdays to achievements, these dishes are crafted with love and care, reflecting the uniqueness of each woman being honored. The delicate balance of flavors mirrors the multifaceted nature of womanhood itself.Moving forward, the chapter explores recipes perfect for gatherings that embrace the spirit of sisterhood. Whether it's a bridal shower, baby shower, or a simple get-together of friends, these culinary creations serve as a communal feast, symbolizing the importance of support and camaraderie among women.The heart of this chapter lies in the exploration of cultural and traditional dishes that pay homage to the diverse roles women play around the world. From timeless classics to modern interpretations, each recipe encapsulates the rich tapestry of global womanhood, fostering a sense of unity through the shared experience of culinary delights.Additionally, the chapter highlights the joy of self-care and indulgence with recipes designed for moments of personal celebration. Whether it's a quiet evening alone or a weekend treat, these dishes provide an opportunity for women to pamper themselves, savoring the pleasures of good food and self-appreciation.As the chapter concludes, it leaves readers with a profound appreciation for the unique journey of womanhood. The recipes presented are not merely culinary creations but expressions of love, empowerment, and celebration, making this chapter a delightful culinary odyssey

dedicated to honoring and cherishing the essence
of being a woman.

Chapter Fourteen
The Art of Meal Planning: Simplifying Healthy Eating

The Art of Meal Planning: Simplifying Healthy EatingIn the intricate dance of our daily lives, the often-overlooked choreography of meal planning takes center stage in Chapter Fourteen. Here, the author skillfully navigates the complexities of balancing nutrition and convenience, unveiling the art of meal planning as a powerful tool for simplifying healthy eating.The chapter begins by demystifying the misconceptions surrounding meal planning, emphasizing its transformative potential for fostering a healthier lifestyle. The author highlights the benefits of strategic meal preparation, from improved portion control to the reduction of food waste. By meticulously laying out the groundwork, readers are equipped with practical tips to seamlessly integrate meal planning into their routines.The narrative delves into the core principles of crafting nutritious and well-balanced meals. It emphasizes the importance of incorporating a variety of food groups, ensuring a spectrum of essential nutrients. The reader is guided through the process of creating personalized meal plans that cater to individual dietary needs and preferences. This tailored approach enhances the sustainability of healthy eating habits, debunking the myth that nutritious meals must sacrifice flavor.The chapter further explores time-saving strategies and kitchen hacks, presenting a repertoire of efficient techniques to streamline meal preparation. From batch cooking to strategic grocery shopping, the author unveils a toolkit that empowers readers to navigate the often-overwhelming landscape of healthy eating with confidence and ease.Throughout the narrative, practical examples and real-life success stories underscore the feasibility of embracing the art of meal planning. By showcasing diverse scenarios and illustrating the positive impact on individuals' lives, the author reinforces the notion that this practice is not an unattainable ideal but an adaptable and rewarding skill.In conclusion, Chapter Fourteen serves as a beacon for those seeking to embark on a journey towards simplified and healthier eating. With a blend of insightful guidance and tangible strategies, readers are not only educated on the art of meal planning but also inspired to make lasting changes that resonate with the rhythm of their lives.

Chapter Fifteen
Kitchen Tips and Tricks: Making Healthier Cooking Effortless

Kitchen Tips and Tricks: Making Healthier Cooking EffortlessIn this enlightening chapter, we delve into a treasure trove of kitchen wisdom, unraveling tips and tricks that effortlessly elevate your cooking endeavors to healthier heights. The kitchen is more than just a place to prepare meals; it's a realm where choices made can significantly impact well-being.One key insight revolves around ingredient swaps. Learn how to seamlessly replace refined sugars with natural sweeteners, turning your guilty pleasures into guilt-free indulgences. Uncover the art of incorporating whole grains, enhancing the nutritional profile of your dishes without compromising on taste. This chapter unravels the secrets of using healthier fats and oils, guiding you towards options that benefit heart health without skimping on flavor.Portion control takes center stage, shedding light on the importance of mindful eating. Discover strategies to balance your plate, ensuring a harmonious blend of proteins, vegetables, and whole grains. Unearth the power of herbs and spices, transforming your meals into culinary delights with added health benefits.Struggling with meal prepping? Fear not, as this chapter provides practical insights into planning and prepping nutritious meals efficiently. From batch cooking to strategic storage, these tips make it a breeze to maintain a healthy diet, even on the busiest of days.The chapter also explores cooking techniques that retain nutrients without sacrificing taste. Dive into the world of steaming, roasting, and sautéing to discover how these methods enhance flavors while preserving the nutritional integrity of your ingredients.Armed with these kitchen hacks, making healthier choices becomes second nature. Whether you're a seasoned chef or a novice in the culinary arts, Chapter Fifteen is your guide to transforming your kitchen into a hub of health and wellness, where every meal is a step towards a more vibrant and balanced lifestyle.

Conclusion

A Culinary Companion for Women's Well-being
In conclusion, the concept of a culinary companion for women's well-being emerges as a holistic approach to nurturing both physical and mental health. Through the exploration of diverse cuisines, nutritional awareness, and mindful eating practices, this culinary journey becomes a powerful ally in fostering well-being.The fusion of taste and nutrition not only satisfies the palate but also contributes to the overall vitality of women. The importance of a balanced diet cannot be overstated, and a culinary companion serves as a guide, promoting wholesome food choices that cater to specific nutritional needs. By embracing a variety of ingredients, rich in essential vitamins and minerals, women can proactively support their health.Moreover, the act of preparing and sharing meals becomes a therapeutic ritual, fostering a sense of connection and community. Cooking serves as a creative outlet, allowing women to express themselves through flavors and textures. This shared experience, whether

with family or friends, cultivates a supportive environment, reinforcing emotional well-being.The culinary companion extends beyond the kitchen, influencing lifestyle choices and encouraging mindfulness. Adopting mindful eating practices brings attention to the present moment, promoting a healthy relationship with food and reducing stress. This mindful approach, when integrated into daily life, has a profound impact on overall mental and emotional equilibrium.In essence, a culinary companion for women's well-being is not merely about sustenance but a celebration of health, creativity, and connection. It empowers women to take charge of their nutritional choices, inspiring a positive relationship with food that echoes through every aspect of their lives. As we savor the richness of diverse cuisines, we simultaneously savor the richness of life, embracing a culinary journey that nourishes body, mind, and soul.

www.ingramcontent.com/pod-product-compliance
Lightning Source LLC
Chambersburg PA
CBHW070957260726
48661CB00007B/2743